STRATEGY FOR WEIGHT LOSS

Wesley M. Newby

Contents

Chapter One

Diet Plan for Losing Weight in Two Weeks

If you want to lose weight in two weeks, a two-week diet plan may help you achieve your goals without requiring a long-term commitment. A two-week diet plan's main premise is that you should consume less calories than you expend. This can only be accomplished by restricting your food consumption, although it is possible to drop up to 20 pounds during this period. This strategy is great for exceptional events like holidays or vacations.

If you want to lose 10 pounds in two weeks, you'll need a larger deficit than if you want to drop 10 pounds in one week. For example, if you want to lose five pounds in a week, you'll need to reduce your maintenance calories by 17,500 calories. This implies that instead of 500 calories per day, you'll need to establish a daily deficit of about 2500.

While losing weight may be a motivating and uplifting experience, it's also vital to realize that stress can make sticking to a diet plan more difficult. Stress has been linked to an increase in food cravings and the storage of fat in the body, according to studies. You may easily lose weight in two weeks if you avoid stressful circumstances and reduce the amount of stress in your life. This is a good option if you want a diet plan that has been proved to work.

Exercising to Lose Weight in Two Weeks is the best way to lose weight in two weeks.

Start with a calorie deficit if you want to lose weight in 2 weeks. To be successful, this calorie restriction must be well-thought-out and balanced. Each exercise should have a maximum of 10 repetitions.

If you're a newbie, though, you might consider adding in some additional sessions to help you become used to the routine and get benefits faster. The most significant weight-loss techniques will be discussed in this post.

Make sure you consume a balanced diet. You should consume less than you burn throughout the first two weeks. It's advisable to aim for a weekly weight loss of 10 pounds, or 5% of your present weight. Make sure you perform three sets of 10 to 12 repetitions every day. In a few weeks, these activities will help you lose at least 10 pounds. Simply complete three sets of ten to twelve repetitions.

Make an effort to concentrate on your exercises. You will lose more weight than you believe if you exercise every day. The key to accomplishing this aim is to concentrate on a training routine that includes a larger number of repetitions and lower body fat percentage. Furthermore, rather of consuming manufactured junk food, you should concentrate on eating real meals. Furthermore, these diets are high in fiber and may aid in the attainment of your objectives.

Meal Plan for Losing Weight in Two Weeks

You may lose six to ten pounds in a month by following a two-week eating regimen. It comes with meals, exercises, and customer service that is available 24 hours a day, seven days a week. In only two weeks, you may lose a lot of weight by following the two-week eating plan. You should make certain lifestyle modifications to get the greatest outcomes, such as eating less calories and drinking less alcohol. You may attain your goal weight in a few of weeks if you stick to a two-week food plan.

You should contact a nutritionist and a doctor before embarking on a new diet. A healthy food plan might be suggested by your doctor. The amount of weight you can shed is determined by a number of variables, including your overall health, underlying medical issues, daily exercise level, and dietary choices. You may locate a food plan that meets your demands and assists you in losing weight quickly by visiting a health specialist.

The 2-week meal plan might help you get started on a healthy, clean diet. The emphasis is on eating more fruits and vegetables and preferring fresh fruits and vegetables than processed snacks. This meal plan is intended to aid weight loss and general wellness. If you stick to this regimen, you'll start losing weight and eating better than you have in the past. You'll feel fantastic and have much less energy than previously!

Chapter Two

Weight Loss Pills that Work in 2 Weeks

While it may seem tough to lose weight in two weeks, it is feasible to do it safely. To reduce weight, you don't have to follow fad diets or use risky drugs. A mix of exercise and proper nutrition is one of the many safe ways to decrease extra fat. However, you should be aware that two weeks is insufficient time to notice significant improvements. Here are some weight-loss techniques that are both safe and effective.

Before you do anything else, be sure you read the label. You shouldn't simply believe the first component on the label. It's better to avoid a product if the components on the label seem to be questionable. Doing your study and selecting a different brand is a better option. If the ingredients on the bottle aren't stated, don't purchase it. Instead, do your homework and make an educated choice. Today's market is flooded with choices.

Before using any weight-loss supplement, be sure you read the label. Some companies may attempt to persuade you to purchase their product by advertising it as the "greatest recipe ever" while concealing potentially dangerous elements. Before purchasing a drug, make sure you do your study and know what's in it. After that, you'll be able to make an educated choice. Accept nothing less than the best! In a few weeks, you'll feel much better and happy.

When picking a diet pill, it is important to read the label. Be aware of companies who claim to have the "greatest" recipe while omitting the potentially dangerous elements. Before deciding on one, you should conduct some study. Also, be sure to read the label of the medication you're thinking about taking. Artificial sweeteners and colorants, among other things, might be contained in certain medicines. It's preferable if you don't take any until you're certain they're safe.

It's important to read the label before using a weight-loss supplement. Some medicines include potentially dangerous chemicals like chitosan, which is derived from lobster and shrimp shells. Chitosan, on the other hand, is insufficient for weight loss. It's better to choose a pill that is free of these chemicals. To locate the greatest diet medication, you may perform your own study.

You should examine the contents on the package of any diet pill before purchasing it. Chitosan, a chemical derived from lobster and shrimp shells, may be included in several tablets. These drugs, on the other hand, have no discernible weight-loss effects. Stimulants, such as caffeine and guarana, are other prominent constituents in diet tablets. It's also a good idea to verify the pill's dose.

You should pay attention to the components on the bottle in addition to reading the label. Some pills claim to have the "greatest ever" formula and health-promoting components. It would be great if you done your homework and learned all there is to know about the pill's contents. Artificial components are used in certain goods, which might have negative consequences. As a result, before purchasing a diet medication, you should always consult a pharmacist. Your doctor will be able to point out the chemicals and inform you how dangerous they are to your health.

You should learn about the components of a diet pill before purchasing it. While many goods claim to be "best of the best," certain consumers may wish to explore for additional components. Caffeine, for example, is included in a lot of weight reduction medicines. However, this is only one of several ingredients that might be harmful. Before buying any product, you should carefully read the ingredients list and compare it to comparable goods. This will guarantee that your diet yields the finest possible outcomes.

Reading the label is the first step in finding the correct diet medication. While some of these items may seem to be helpful to your health, you should check the contents to see whether they are.

While certain tablets are safer than others, you should always see a pharmacist before taking any medication. Never purchase a medication without first contacting a physician. Taking a medicine that doesn't work is the worst.

Chapter Three

Is it Possible to Lose Significant Weight in Just Two Weeks?

The subject of whether or not it is possible to reduce significant weight in two weeks has long been debated. Underlying health issues, daily activity level, and dietary choices are just a few of the elements that influence weight reduction pace. There are various strategies for losing considerable quantities of body fat rapidly, fortunately. Some of the most efficient methods for losing weight are listed here. This post will look at some of the most efficient ways to lose weight quickly.

Eating right and exercising are the initial steps to reducing weight rapidly. Losing one to two pounds each week should be the objective. You'll most likely drop a few pounds each week if you start at a healthy weight. One to two pounds per week is a reasonable weight-loss target. While this is more quickly than most individuals can reach, reducing your calorie intake or exercising less is not a smart option. It's possible that you'll acquire more weight than you expected.

It's a tall order to lose one to two pounds each week. The average person may lose one to two pounds every week, which is a significant amount of weight. The outcomes of a diet and exercise regimen, on the other hand, will differ from person to person. Even if your strategy works for some people, it isn't right for everyone. You may shed a few pounds in a week, but your physique will most likely change dramatically in the following weeks.

While a week or two may seem like a long time to you, your outcomes will most certainly differ. If you follow a diet and exercise plan, you should lose a couple of pounds every week, which is a reasonable target for most people. Regardless, how much weight you lose will be determined by your size, degree of activity, and daily calorie expenditure. It's not a good idea to attempt to shed more weight than this since it might harm your health.

Is Running a Good Way to Lose Weight in Two Weeks?

What is the maximum amount of weight I can lose in two weeks if I run? It depends entirely on the circumstances. It takes 3,500 calories to burn one pound of fat. Running for two hours each day, on the other hand, may help you lose half a pound in a week. The majority of individuals consume more calories than they burn because they overeat. As a result, they burn less calories at the start of their activity. As a consequence, individuals seem to be more tireder than they really are.

A calorie deficit is necessary for weight loss. This implies you have to burn more calories than you consume. You should consume less calories in order to do this. Protein-rich meals are essential for feeling satisfied.

It's also ideal if you don't eat too much. Before beginning a running program, it's a good idea to follow a rigorous food plan.

A healthy diet should be part of your running program. Small meals are required, and high-calorie foods should be avoided. Rather, consume fewer high-calorie, high-fat items and more veggies and nutritious grains. You should also have a protein-rich and satiating post-run meal. Knowing how much to eat each day is also crucial. If you're a beginner runner, you may estimate how many calories you'll require using a simple calculator.

Running speeds up your metabolism and increases your hunger. When you're hungry after a run, it's easy to overeat. To overcome this issue, eat a high-protein, appropriately portioned post-run meal. This will provide you with the necessary energy to complete your next run. When you're ready to start jogging, start with a basic routine and see how it works.

A nutritious diet, in addition to the advantages of jogging, will aid in weight loss. It's critical to eat nutrient-dense meals. It is not advisable to lose weight by eating a high-carbohydrate diet. Stick to a high-protein diet if you want to lose weight. Running will keep you small and fit, even if it isn't the cheapest strategy to reduce weight.

Running for as least two weeks may usually help you lose a pound of weight. You need to consume less than you burn to lose a pound of fat. It's important to follow a diet plan and eat a healthy post-run meal. This will assist your muscles recuperate by keeping your blood sugar levels in check. For the first two weeks, it's advisable to have a calorie deficit of 500 calories each day.

Running can help you lose weight in a healthy way, but you need also eat well. Burning 3500 calories each week is a decent rule of thumb for losing a pound per week. Higher-density muscle tissue must replace a pound of fat. Burning 500 calories per day is required to lose a pound of fat. At least one pound of fat should be burned every week.

When it comes to weight reduction, running is a wonderful workout to try. It's a great way to burn calories and improve your cardiovascular health. It's not just about how many calories you burn, however. Your weight is influenced by a number of things. Diet, hormones, heredity, and general lifestyle are all factors to consider. Even if you run often, it's important to manage your expectations.

While exercise might help you lose weight, eating healthy is as important. You will not lose weight by drinking extra water throughout your run. Adding to your overall body weight by drinking additional water after a run is a waste of time. After your exercise, a nutritious post-run meal will aid in your recovery. It will help you maintain a healthy blood sugar level and provide your muscles the nutrients they need to repair themselves. You may begin jogging at your neighborhood park or gym in two weeks and notice benefits.

Chapter Four

Is it possible to lose weight in two weeks if you exercise?

People lose weight for a variety of reasons, including health, body form, and just for the sake of having fun. While there are a variety of methods for achieving your objectives, reducing weight quickly is typically the best choice for you and your body. Diet medicines and procedures are used by certain individuals, but a diet and exercise regimen is a healthier and more long-term option. Here are some pointers to help you get started and stay on track:

When attempting to lose weight quickly, cutting calories is one of the most crucial things to remember. A typical guy requires 2,500 calories per day, thus eliminating 500 calories every day for a week will result in a loss of 3,500 calories. To lose 10 pounds in two weeks, a person needs burn five pounds each week, or 17,500 calories less than usual. This isn't a simple task, but if you can commit to it for a few weeks, you can accomplish it.

You'll need to consume less than your typical maintenance amount if you want to lose up to 20 pounds in two weeks. That does not, however, imply that you must abstain entirely. Just keep in mind that a higher deficit implies you'll burn more calories than you consume. To lose weight in two weeks, you'll need to eat roughly 17500 calories less each day than you normally do. This implies that instead of 500 calories per day, you'll need to consume 2,000 calories less each day.

You'll need to expend 17,500 calories less than usual to drop 10 pounds in two weeks. That's a lot of calories, but it's not out of the question. In only a few weeks, you'll be able to lose the additional weight by combining the correct activities with a healthy lifestyle. So, if you want to lose 10 pounds in two weeks, begin by reducing your calorie intake.

Cutting calories is the most effective approach of losing 20 pounds in two weeks. It's ideal if you can burn more calories than you consume. You'll need to limit your daily consumption if you want to drop 10 pounds in two weeks with exercise. This entails eating less and consuming less calories in general. You might drop up to 10 pounds in two weeks.

Calorie restriction is the secret to reducing weight in two weeks without exercising. You'll need to cut your calorie consumption by roughly a third if you want to drop around 10 pounds in two weeks. To burn as much fat in two weeks, do three sets of workouts at least three times each week. You'll be amazed at how rapidly you lose weight if you can accomplish this.

Cutting your calorie consumption is the most effective strategy to lose 10 pounds in two weeks without exercising. A daily calorie requirement is around 2,500 calories. As a consequence, a daily calorie reduction of 500 calories will result in a three-pound weight loss. With adequate exercise and a nutritious diet, this weight is readily achieved. You may drop 10 pounds in two weeks by combining a nutritious diet with a regular exercise regimen.

You must cut your calorie consumption by 20% to lose 20 pounds in two weeks without exercising. You want to burn more calories than you eat. This may be done safely if you consume a balanced diet and exercise more. You can also eat less calories. You may drop 10 pounds in only two weeks if you workout every day. You will acquire weight if you eat more calories than your body requires.

You must lower your calorie consumption if you want to drop more than 10 pounds in two weeks. A man's daily calorie requirement is 2,500. A weekly weight loss of three pounds may be achieved by reducing calories by 500 per day. You must reduce your food consumption by more than half in order to drop 10 pounds in two weeks. Furthermore, if you want to lose additional weight, you'll need to reduce your fat intake by roughly 50%.

Is it possible to shed pounds in two weeks?

When considering whether or not you can lose weight in two weeks, keep in mind that you must adjust your lifestyle as well as your nutrition. While two weeks may seem to be a small period of time, it might be the ideal time to observe effects. If you want to lose weight safely and permanently, follow a healthy, balanced diet and exercise regimen. You'll be on your way to achieving your weight-loss objectives in no time if you follow these suggestions.

A calorie deficit is the key to reducing weight rapidly. Although this may seem to be a significant amount of time, the typical guy need roughly 2,500 calories each day to maintain life and keep his body working correctly. Sticking to a healthy and long-term weight-loss regimen is crucial to success. You may concentrate on developing a new healthy lifestyle after you've discovered an excellent diet and exercise routine.

Following a healthy diet and exercise program is one of the most important things to keep in mind when trying to lose weight. Unlike fad diets, this strategy is both safe and healthful, making it simpler to stick to your weight-loss objectives. It's critical to stick to your diet and exercise plan to avoid regaining weight. It's essential to keep things basic and regular when starting a new fitness regimen, since sticking to a pattern over time is much simpler.

It is important to get advice from a doctor or a certified nutritionist before beginning a weight-loss program in order to maintain a healthy lifestyle and diet. If you have a lot of additional weight to lose, you may be able to shed 20 pounds in a few weeks. It may take longer to lose tiny amounts of weight. Additionally, reducing weight in two weeks is hard for everyone.

It's simple to lose weight quickly by changing your diet. Generally, eating less than you burn is a good idea. It is possible to reduce weight by consuming less calories than you need. You'll be more effective in reducing weight if you consume a higher-calorie diet as your aim. High-calorie, high-fat, or low-calorie meals should also be avoided.

It is not advisable to lose weight quickly. You will lose weight and not obtain adequate nutrients if you attempt to decrease your calories in half. Each day, you'll need to consume fewer than 200 calories. You should also consume at least 5,000 calories each day. It's advisable to strive for a weekly weight loss of at least 2 pounds. If you stick to this strategy, you'll see visible improvements in two weeks.

You may lose weight by burning more calories than you eat if you follow a healthy diet plan. It does not necessitate a major dietary change. Fat cells will be lost in the same amount of time as if you ate a normal diet. It's a terrific technique to tone up and look better. It's also a great method to stay in shape. So don't let a healthy diet pass you by in the next two weeks.

It's important to remember that everyone's weight loss will be different. A calorie deficit is necessary for a healthy weight loss plan. You should also be aware of your current health status as well as any underlying health issues. Making drastic dietary changes without consulting a doctor is not a good idea. Weight loss entails altering one's lifestyle and eating habits in addition to losing fat. How quickly you lose weight is influenced by a number of other factors.

When you're trying to lose weight, you'll want to cut down on your calorie intake. Setting up a calorie deficit and balancing your diet and exercise are the keys to success. You'll have a harder time losing weight if you don't consume as many calories as you should. If you want to lose weight in two weeks, go for high-intensity exercises that will help you burn more calories.

Chapter Five

How Can Running Help Me Lose Weight in 2 Weeks?

Many people are unsure if running can aid in weight loss. This is a common query, particularly among runners who are new to the sport. Running, on the other hand, can help you burn a lot of calories, which can help you lose weight. It's important to remember, however, that losing weight is about more than just burning calories. It's also crucial to understand how your body responds to different types of exercise, diet, and hormone levels.

When you run on a regular basis, you can burn up to 300 calories per mile. This is the extra oxygen consumption that occurs after a vigorous workout. You should lose one or two pounds per week. This is an excellent place to begin your weight-loss journey. Running at least three times per week is also essential. This will assist you in burning more fat than usual.

Running helps you burn calories by increasing your metabolism. Running is a good option if you're looking for a quick way to lose weight because it also builds strength and endurance. You'll be well on your way if you combine this exercise with proper nutrition, strength training, and increased fitness. You'll lose weight and keep it off without going hungry! Running has numerous advantages, even if you are new to the sport.

Making good food choices is the most effective way to lose weight while running. Creating a 500-calorie deficit every day is the most effective way to lose weight. After a 30-minute run, you'll be able to burn fat for two days. Try walking or biking instead of running if you haven't already. This will help you lose weight more quickly, and the exercise will help you feel more energized.

Running increases your metabolism, so keep that in mind. This translates to more energy and a longer feeling of fullness. You'll be less likely to overeat as a result of it.

Aside from running, smart eating can aid weight loss by lowering calorie intake. If you're already overweight or obese, limiting your carb intake after a workout is a good idea.

Is Walking a Good Way to Lose Weight in Two Weeks?

Walking has a number of advantages, the most important of which is that it increases cardiovascular endurance.

While aerobic exercise is important for heart health, walking requires more energy, so you should push yourself to work at a faster pace. While walking burns calories, you should increase the distance you walk to burn more. Strength and resistance training can also be beneficial to your overall health.

You must ensure that you can stick to the plan and maintain the same level of exercise, as with most exercise routines. You must maintain a moderate calorie deficit to lose weight, so eat a well-balanced diet. Brush your arms across your body while walking with your arms bent 90 degrees. Avoid overstretched or hunched legs, as they add more calories than a balanced diet. Walking regularly will strengthen your legs and lower your blood pressure, in addition to burning more calories.

Creating a calorie deficit is essential for rapid weight loss. To achieve long-term weight loss, it is critical to stick to your plan. The average adult loses a pound per week, but those who weigh more than 200 pounds will find it more difficult. It's critical to set a reasonable goal for yourself when it comes to walking, so start small and work your way up to a healthier lifestyle! The more weight you lose the longer you stick to your walking schedule.

The most common cause of obesity is poor eating habits. They eat more than they expend. Eat a well-balanced diet that includes whole grains, fresh fruit, vegetables, beans, lentils, nuts, seeds, and other healthy foods to create a calorie deficit. Starting with an activity that you enjoy is the best way to begin walking. Set a daily or weekly challenge for yourself and see how well you can stick to it.

How Can I Lose Weight Without Exercising in Two Weeks?

"How can I lose weight in two weeks without exercising?" is a question that many people are asking. Many people want to lose weight for a variety of reasons, ranging from improved health to a different body shape. Some people simply want to lose weight for the sake of it! You can lose weight using a variety of methods, such as surgeries and pills. A diet and lifestyle change, on the other hand, is a more long-term and healthy method of weight loss. Here are a few pointers to get you going.

Alcohol and sugary drinks should be avoided. Alcohol has been shown in a number of studies to increase calorie burn and contribute to obesity. Fortunately, there are a slew of other options for losing weight without adding a single calorie to your daily intake. The egg diet is a good way to lose weight without gaining weight. Make sure you drink only water or zero-calorie beverages, and eat breakfast and lunch every day. It would also be ideal if you ate a well-balanced meal that included plenty of fruits and vegetables.

Remember that losing weight is never an easy task, regardless of which method you use. Patience and a balanced lifestyle are required. Don't be swayed by the promise of 20 pounds lost in two weeks. In the long run, it might not be sustainable. It's important to remember that dieting by itself will not get you the results you want. Combine a healthy diet with exercise if you want to lose weight quickly.

Weight loss should last at least two weeks in order to be effective. During this time, you should incorporate lifestyle changes to help you maintain a healthy weight. Making these changes can help you reach a healthy weight in two weeks. You'll be surprised at how quickly you can shed pounds. This is an effective method for maintaining a healthy metabolism and a slim figure. You'll get the results you want with a two-week fast!

Before attempting to lose weight in two weeks, you should consult with your doctor. While you can lose weight without exercising, you should follow the rules and consult your doctor. This method should not be attempted if you are not in good health, as it may harm your health. Furthermore, before beginning this program, make sure you follow your doctor's instructions.

A change in your diet and way of life can also help your health. Water and unsweetened coffee should be your only beverages. A 12-ounce glass of red wine and a 12-ounce whole-milk latte each have 150 calories. As a result, it's critical to stay away from alcohol while on a weight-loss diet.

Furthermore, when trying to lose weight, it's always a good idea to think about your dietary preferences. A qualified nutritionist should be consulted as well.

There are numerous methods for losing weight that do not require physical activity. You should eat a healthy diet and limit your intake of unhealthy foods in general. You should also keep your alcohol consumption to a minimum. It will also increase your risk of developing health problems and will not aid in long-term weight loss. Alcohol consumption can be harmful to your health. As a result, no alcohol should be consumed during the two-week diet.

You should think about your dietary choices in addition to exercising. A common misconception is that weight loss can be achieved solely through a diet. In reality, a healthy, long-term result will not come from diet alone. A healthy lifestyle will help you lose weight and keep it off. And don't expect to notice a significant change in your body size in less than two weeks.

Before attempting a diet and exercise plan, it is critical to speak with a medical professional or a qualified nutritionist. Losing a pound per day is a reasonable target. Aim for 500 to 1,000 calories per day to lose one pound per week. You can lose up to two pounds a week without exercising if you do it this way. A low-calorie diet will not help you if you have a health problem.

How Can a Keto Diet Help You Lose Weight in Two Weeks?

On the ketogenic diet, how do you lose weight in two weeks? It's not impossible, but you'll need to stick to a few rules and avoid a few blunders. Week one should not be spent counting macros or drastically reducing calories. It's critical to stick to a low-calorie diet for two weeks. It's best if you set a weekly weight loss goal of a few pounds. It would be best if you followed your weight-loss plan gradually.

Although the link between obesity and cancer is debatable, it is well established that having a high body fat percentage raises the risk of certain cancers. Higher levels of body fat have been linked to breast, colorectal, and kidney cancer. Endometrial cancer is more common in women who are overweight. Weight loss necessitates a caloric deficit, which means eating fewer calories than you burn.

On the ketogenic diet, gradually lowering your calorie intake is the key to losing weight. Although weight loss may be slow and steady at first, a pound of weight loss per week should be the goal. Then you can start over. Weight loss will continue to be gradual after the first week, but you'll need to eat less to keep the deficit going. You can resume your normal eating habits once you reach your desired weight.

You might lose 1-2 pounds per week if you have a faster metabolism. However, your weight loss may slow slightly, and you'll need to eat fewer calories than before to maintain your current weight loss rate. Stick to the diet plan and drop a few pounds per week if you want to lose weight quickly. Your outcomes will satisfy you. You will lose weight in two weeks if you stick with it.

The weight loss will slow down after you've started the ketogenic diet. It will then begin to slow. As your metabolism slows, you'll need to eat fewer calories to keep the deficit going.

Your weight will stay consistent at 1-2 pounds per week after the first week. To keep your weight at the same level, you'll need to continue to eat less. Your body will then become accustomed to the new diet.

The ketogenic diet will help you lose at least two pounds in two weeks. For this, you'll need a lot of water. You should also remember that fat loss will continue in the coming weeks. You'll be eating less than usual once you start the ketogenic diet. You should aim for a weekly weight loss of one to two pounds.

You'll probably lose 1-2 pounds in a week, despite the fact that you'll be eating more than you require. You will be on the road to a healthier body if you lose more than two pounds per week. For a few weeks after the first week, you'll feel lighter and more energetic. If you're having trouble losing weight, try fasting for a few days and then sticking to your diet.

You shouldn't expect to lose all of your weight on a ketogenic diet. To avoid overeating or undereating, as with any diet, you should keep track of your weight fluctuations. During the first two weeks, you may experience some weight fluctuation, but your goal is to lose one to two pounds per week. Even in three days or less, you can lose weight.

It's possible to lose weight in two weeks if you're on a ketogenic diet. The fat-burning mechanism of the ketogenic diet allows you to feel fuller faster and for longer. You'll also be lighter than you've ever been. Despite this, the first week may leave you feeling sluggish and tired. Fasting for a week will aid in the recovery of the flu and increase your energy levels.

Chapter Six

Without Exercise, How to Lose Weight in 2 Weeks

Reducing your caloric intake is the most effective way to lose weight in two weeks without exercise. Without exercising, this is the most effective way to lose 20 pounds in two weeks. If you want to lose weight, you should cut down on your calorie intake. Cutting back on what you eat is the best way to achieve this. How do you go about doing this, though? To begin, you must be conscious of your eating patterns. You will gain more fat and lose more weight than necessary if you eat too much.

Drinks should be limited if you're trying to lose weight. You only have two options: water or unsweetened coffee. Red wine has 125 calories, as does a 12-ounce latte with whole milk. This means that during the two-week diet, you should avoid these beverages. It's recommended that you include a drink after a meal in your daily calorie intake to avoid weight loss.

If you're thinking about going on a no-carb diet, you'll want to keep your carb intake low. The goal is to restore normal protein and carbohydrate levels in your body before gradually introducing new foods. Remember to include vegetables, lean proteins, and healthy fats in your diet. You can lose 20 pounds in two weeks if you stick to this plan. Remember, before beginning any diet, you should always consult your doctor.

Consult a qualified nutritionist or doctor if you want to lose weight quickly without exercising. Several factors, including your current health, any underlying medical conditions, and your dietary preferences, will determine the best method for you. So, before starting any fast weight-loss diet, make sure to talk to your doctor.

Sticking to a healthy diet and a balanced exercise program are the only ways to lose weight quickly and safely.

How to Exercise at Home to Lose Weight in 2 Weeks

The egg diet is a popular weight-loss plan. Two or three eggs per day are required. Then zero-calorie drinks like water or fruit juice would be ideal. A balanced diet should also include whole-grain bread, fruit, salad, chicken, and vegetables. The best part is that you can see results in as little as two weeks if you stick to the diet.

To lose weight quickly, however, you must first understand your current fitness level, underlying health issues, and dietary preferences. You must be honest about your fitness level and time commitment, regardless of which type of exercise program you choose. Only if your schedule and fitness level allow for a two-week exercise plan, will it be effective. Try a different diet if you can't stick to the plan.

A low-carb diet can help you lose weight quickly, but you must be honest about your current fitness level before beginning your new exercise routine. To make sure your diet plan is the right one for you, ask yourself a few questions. If you're in good overall health and don't have any underlying medical conditions, talk to your doctor and nutritionist. A two-week plan will help you determine how much weight you can lose safely.

Sugary beverages should be avoided if you want to shed up to 20 pounds in two weeks. The calorie content of alcohol is high. As a result, it's critical to abstain from consuming any alcohol for two weeks. You should also think about how much energy you use on a daily basis. If you decide to keep drinking alcohol, make sure to include it in your exercise routine. You should consult a medical professional or a dietitian if you want to lose weight quickly. Remember that losing 20 pounds in two weeks is a difficult goal to achieve if you don't eat well and exercise regularly.

You should consult with your doctor before beginning a new exercise regimen. Whether or not you can lose weight in two weeks will be determined by your health and fitness level. You should also consider how much time you have available for exercise. It's a good idea to consult a qualified nutritionist and a nutritionist if you're unsure about how to lose weight in two weeks.

It's critical to assess your fitness level before beginning any exercise program. If you're not in great shape, a qualified health care professional can help you figure out what plan is best for you. While an exercise program can help you lose up to 20 pounds, it's important not to overdo it. It will only cause you frustration in the long run. This is why the most effective exercise program is one that is tailored to your specific objectives.

It is best to exercise regularly to lose twenty pounds. However, if you only eat carbohydrates, you won't be able to do so. If you want to lose weight, it's best if you eat plenty of protein. To stay hydrated and get the nutrients you need, you should drink water in addition to eating healthy foods.

In addition, increasing your intake of healthy fats will help you burn more calories.

Consult your doctor and a qualified nutritionist before beginning a new diet. The amount of weight you lose in two weeks is determined by a variety of factors, including your overall health, underlying medical conditions, activity levels, and dietary preferences. It's not easy to lose weight, but with the right strategy, you can do it. You can lose weight in just two weeks if you follow these recommendations.

You should speak with a qualified nutritionist before beginning any diet plan. The weight loss requirements of your body vary. Before starting any diet, it's a good idea to think about your lifestyle and eating habits. You can start your two-week workout program once you've decided which diet to follow. Starting a routine that allows you to lose up to 20 pounds in two weeks is ideal.

Exercise for Weight Loss in 2 Weeks

Working out is a tried and true method for shedding pounds. Drinking plenty of water, cutting calories, and including healthy fats in your diet are some other options. Here are some weight-loss tips from fitness experts. Staying active and eating well are key to losing weight quickly. You'll be slimmer and healthier in no time if you follow these guidelines. Then, to stay motivated, follow these suggestions.

If you're serious about losing weight in a few weeks, you'll need to start at the beginning. Even if you're too tired to exercise, you must be prepared to do so every day. It will be much easier to lose weight in the first few days. Losing weight after a few weeks, however, will be difficult. To accomplish this, you must develop an unbreakable mindset and stick to the program.

You should be motivated to change your lifestyle if you want to lose weight in two weeks. Because stress affects your metabolism, it can make losing weight more difficult. Stress makes your body store more fat in addition to making you crave junk food. As a result, rapid weight loss is extremely difficult. You must first be patient and committed in order to achieve your goal. After that, you can begin exercising and eating a nutritious diet.

It is critical to realize that burning 2,000 calories per day is nearly impossible. Furthermore, dropping 10 pounds in two weeks is no easy task. It takes dedication and a never-say-die attitude. Losing weight in two weeks, like any other endeavor, requires developing long-term healthy habits. Exercises that burn the required number of calories should be chosen. Before beginning any exercise routine, be realistic about your body's capabilities.

Chapter Seven

Natural Weight Loss in Two Weeks

There are many ways to lose weight, but if you're looking to lose weight quickly, a natural approach is the best option. Changing one's lifestyle is one way to go about it. You'll need to cut out processed foods, eat more fruits and vegetables, and drink less soda. A natural method will work best for you if you want to lose 20 pounds in two weeks. It's also a lot healthier than the alternatives.

The key to losing weight naturally is to reduce the amount of salt you eat. The more salt you eat, the easier it is to gain it back. In just two weeks, eliminating salt from your diet is an excellent way to reduce your caloric intake. You'll feel fuller and more energetic in the end. The best way to lose weight naturally is to eat less and exercise more. You can burn fat more efficiently by avoiding refined and processed foods.

While losing weight isn't difficult, a natural diet can help you lose weight faster and more easily than a conventional diet. It's important to keep in mind that a natural weight-loss plan won't help you lose all of your weight in two weeks. However, it will hasten the fat-burning procedure. In a couple of weeks, you'll notice significant changes in your body. You can easily lose weight using this method.

Your metabolism will work overtime to burn excess calories when you're exercising. You'll feel more energetic. You'll also burn more fat. The best way to lose weight in two weeks without working out is to reduce your calorie intake. Keeping a diet low in calories will help you burn more fat. If you're eating too many calories, you'll quickly gain more weight.

In addition to exercising and cutting calories, you should also limit your saturated and trans fats intake. The more saturated fat you have, the more likely you will gain. To avoid these problems, cut down on salt. This simple step will help you lose excess weight. However, if you're not in a hurry to lose weight, you can try the fasting method. But it will not burn all of the fat in your body.

Exercise-Based Weight Loss in 2 Weeks

If you're trying to figure out how to lose weight in two weeks, keep in mind that it's a challenging task. Losing the desired weight necessitates a lot of effort and commitment. There are a variety of elements to consider, which makes it much more difficult. To begin, reduce your calorie intake. This is the most crucial aspect of weight loss.

Aim to burn at least 2,000 calories every day. It's wise to remember that losing 10 pounds in two weeks is practically difficult. It would be ideal if you approached your program with enthusiasm. Work hard and make daily objectives for yourself. It's time to form healthy habits after you've accomplished your objectives. Your fitness level, space availability, and energy level all influence the optimal workout for weight loss. Working within your constraints is the key.

To lose weight quickly, you must change your diet. You must make a deliberate effort to lower your daily calorie intake. You'll lose weight faster if you expend more calories. To lose weight and live a healthy lifestyle, you'll need a diet that enables you to minimize calories while also increasing your activity level. However, if you want to reduce weight faster, you should seek the advice of a fitness professional.

When it comes to exercise, the harder you work out, the more calories you'll burn. Because weight reduction is simpler at the beginning than at the finish, it is best to start a new exercise regimen gently and gradually. By the way, the workout plan you choose should be based on your physical condition as well as the amount of space you have accessible. Keep in mind that you should only exercise to your greatest ability in order to burn the most calories.

Exercise at Home to Lose Weight in 2 Weeks

The first step to reducing weight in two weeks with at-home exercise is to reduce stress. You must remove stress from your life since it is proven to induce hunger and snack cravings. Regular exercise is the most effective strategy to alleviate stress. Over 1,000 calories may be burned in only an hour or two of exercise every day. Regular exercises can also help you lose weight by strengthening your body's fat-fighting resilience.

Cutting calories is the second strategy for losing weight in two weeks with home exercise. A typical male requires roughly 2,500 calories per day, thus cutting 500 calories per day would result in 3,500 calories burned each week. This is one pound of fat, therefore if you want to lose 10 pounds in two weeks, attempt to reduce your calorie intake by five pounds each week. This implies you'll have to lose up to 5 pounds per week.

The next recommendation is to alter your way of living. Limit your fat consumption to roughly 200 grams per day by eating a diet high in vegetables and fruits. It will boost your metabolism and suppress your hunger, allowing you to shed more pounds than you ever imagined. In addition, you should cut your calorie consumption in half to lose weight as quickly as possible. However, you should be aware that this method demands discipline and dedication, and you should always seek the advice of a fitness specialist before starting any diet or exercise regimen.

Cutting down on your calorie consumption is the greatest way to lose 20 pounds in two weeks with workout at home. It's important to remember that if you expend more calories than you consume, you may lose weight. You'll be able to attain your target in two weeks if you cut your calorie consumption by at least half. Just make sure you're dedicated and follow through on your plans.

Without Exercise, How to Lose Weight in 2 Weeks

Without exercising, 20 pounds might be lost in two weeks. This is the best time to shed pounds. It's important to consume fewer calories than you expend. You'll be able to do this by restricting your consumption. However, getting there in that time frame may be difficult, and you'll need to be really driven. Some lifestyle adjustments that will aid weight loss in two weeks are listed below.

You've decided to stay away from alcoholic beverages. While unsweetened coffee or water may leave you feeling full, a 12-ounce glass of alcohol carries roughly 150 calories. So you should abstain from consuming any alcohol for the next two weeks. However, you must consider how much energy you need to maintain your present weight and level of exercise. The most crucial weight-loss guideline is to follow this rule. This diet also encourages good eating habits and a slim body.

Before beginning any new diet or fitness regimen, you should contact with a licensed nutritionist or physician. It's important to keep in mind that this procedure is only appropriate for persons who have major health issues or are obese. Aside from your general health and degree of daily exercise. Also, before beginning any weight-loss regimen, be sure to check your doctor. To avoid major consequences, it is best to take a medication that has been given by a doctor.

A good diet may help you lose weight in as little as two weeks, but you should always get medical advice before embarking on a diet. Consult a dietitian before embarking on a new weight-loss strategy if you have any health issues. For a healthy lifestyle, the appropriate nutrition is necessary. However, if you don't eat well and exercise regularly, reducing weight is a difficult process. To lose weight rapidly and securely, you need follow a rigorous eating plan.

2 Week Workout to Lose Weight

If you're looking for a quick way to lose weight in two weeks, consider making a few basic lifestyle modifications. These modifications will improve the quality of your diet and make portion management simpler. Drinking enough of water before meals will make you feel full, which can help you lose weight quickly. Furthermore, eating fewer meals will increase your energy levels.

A exercise may help you reduce extra pounds in addition to the obvious health advantages. Losing one to two pounds each week would be beneficial. For instance, throughout this period, you should aim to lose four pounds altogether. It's impossible to lose much more. However, you may lose weight in two weeks by following a few simple guidelines. You'll be on your road to a healthier, leaner physique if you stick to these suggestions.

Allow time for your body to adjust to the increased intensity of your exercises. Make sure you rest in between circuits and aim for ten repetitions each exercise. Remember that although this may seem to be a lot, it will really help you lose at least 10 pounds in two weeks. You can always include some cardio. You should, however, begin a fresh weight-loss regimen for the greatest outcomes.

Second, your daily calorie intake should be reduced. Without exercising, this is the most efficient method to reduce weight in two weeks. It's easy to understand why. You will lose weight if you expend more calories than you take in. And the only way to do it is to eat less. Reduce your calorie intake to lose weight. So, start today's fitness journey by reducing your food intake.

You must raise your daily calorie deficit if you want to drop ten pounds in two weeks. Losing 10 pounds in two weeks is possible with a weekly calorie deficit of two thousand calories.

However, if you want to drop 10 pounds in two weeks, don't go beyond this amount.

Furthermore, carbohydrates and sugary meals should be consumed in moderation. Your calorie consumption will be reduced as a result.

How to Lose Weight in 2 Weeks will teach you how to lose weight quickly.

Many individuals want to reduce weight in two weeks but are unable to maintain a consistent program. If this describes you, there are a number of fast and safe strategies to reduce weight. When attempting to lose weight rapidly, the most essential thing to remember is to stay on track. There is no one-size-fits-all approach to shedding pounds. Here are 20 tried-and-true strategies for losing weight in only two weeks. Following these guidelines will allow you to lose as much weight as you want in a week.

We want to see results as soon as possible, which is the most typical motivation for rapid weight loss. However, quick weight reduction is unhealthy for your body. Sticking to a well-balanced diet and avoiding processed foods is the best method to lose weight safely. You may begin your program right now and get results in as little as two weeks. Keep in mind that processed sugars, such as those found in soda, bread, and sweets, must be avoided. While a calorie deficit may seem to be unattainable, it is not. You will notice significant improvements in your fitness objectives within days if you minimize your use of processed sugars.

When it comes to losing weight in two weeks, there are a few factors to consider. You may, for example, be attending the wedding of a high school acquaintance. She invited you to be her maid of honor and had a dress made for you that was too large for you. You still need to reduce weight to make the big day, even if it's just two weeks away. It's crucial to keep in mind that reducing weight isn't tough. Finding a healthy weight reduction program that you can follow to is the greatest approach to drop extra pounds. You should avoid starvation and instead choose a diet that will provide you with the energy and stamina you need to stay on track. You'll have a better chance of keeping the weight off after you've lost it if you do it this way.

Making a nutritious diet is the first step in reducing weight quickly. The most common cause of weight loss in two weeks is refined sugars. Refined sweets don't help you lose weight. Reduce your intake of refined carbohydrates, which are high in calories. Limiting sugar and carbohydrates can give you benefits in as little as two weeks. You'll be more satiated and generally healthier if you consume complete, lean proteins and whole carbohydrates.

How to Lose Weight in 2 Weeks at Home

Try these three simple weight-loss methods if you're seeking for a quick approach to reduce weight. You may achieve your goal of reducing one to two pounds every week by making lifestyle changes. The greatest thing is that you don't even need to leave your house to accomplish it. You can perform them even if you don't have access to a professional. Continue reading to understand more about these three adjustments in lifestyle.

Losing weight quickly requires a balanced diet and frequent exercise. In two weeks, you can lose 20 pounds with a no-carb diet and a few additional methods. To lose weight, you must maintain a calorie deficit. The two most efficient approaches to lose twenty pounds in two weeks are to reduce your daily calorie intake and increase your level of physical activity.

Calorie reduction is the quickest approach to reduce weight. Water and unsweetened coffee are healthy options, but red wine and a 12-ounce latte with full milk are calorie-dense. For two weeks, you should abstain from alcoholic drinks or restrict yourself to two glasses each day. If you want to consume alcohol, remember to account for the calories in your daily energy needs.

Cutting calories is the most effective approach to lose weight in two weeks without exercise. The easiest strategy to lose 20 pounds in two weeks is to eat less calories than you consume. You lose weight when you eat less calories than you burn.

If you just want to drop a few pounds, however, you should get medical advice before attempting this regimen. Only if you have a lot of extra weight will this rapid procedure work.

Setting realistic objectives is critical if you're seeking for the quickest approach to lose 20 pounds. You should aim for a weekly weight loss of one to two pounds, and you should be prepared to put in the effort to achieve it. It's important to keep in mind that dropping too much weight might be dangerous and difficult to maintain. If you're having trouble losing weight, start gently and gradually gain the momentum you'll need to achieve your objective.

Find out how to lose weight in two weeks without exercising.

You can learn to lose weight in two weeks without exercising by adopting a few basic lifestyle adjustments, regardless of your current weight or fitness level. These little adjustments can help you reach your weight-loss goals. To lose weight quickly, use these strategies. You may drop up to 20 pounds in only two weeks by making the necessary lifestyle modifications. Here are a few easy weight-loss ideas. You'll notice benefits quickly if you cut your regular calorie consumption.

Start a low-calorie diet: If you want to reduce weight quickly, consider the egg diet. Only zero-calorie beverages, three short meals each day, and two or three eggs are included in this diet. You may also have fruits and vegetables, as well as whole-wheat bread and cooked eggs on occasion. To keep your metabolism active and maintain your goal weight, you may wish to start a regular exercising routine.

Limiting your alcohol consumption is crucial to lose weight quickly. Despite the fact that this may seem to be detrimental, it may help you succeed. A glass of wine with 12 ounces has 125 calories, while a cup of coffee with full milk has 150 calories. You should start counting calories in addition to avoiding alcohol. You can even monitor your calorie consumption with calorie-tracking apps.

Before beginning a weight-loss program, see a dietitian or doctor. Several variables, including your general health and underlying health issues, will influence the sort of food and activity you select. Your weight reduction pace may be affected by factors such as your daily exercise level and food habits. Consulting with a skilled nutritionist may help you identify the right diet for you.

There are a variety of reasons why a weight-loss strategy may not work for you, so consult your doctor before starting any exercise program.

2 Week Workout to Lose Weight

With the appropriate diet and fitness regimen, you may drop 20 pounds in two weeks without exercising. It's worth noting, though, that losing weight requires burning more calories than you eat. To lower your calorie consumption, you must also limit your regular meals and snacks. You must limit your alcohol and caffeine intake in addition to exercising.

As a consequence, weight reduction will be quick and simple.

You'll have to consume more than 2,500 calories every day to shed 10 pounds in two weeks. This implies you'll need to consume 17,500 calories less per week than your maintenance amount. To put it another way, to lose the same amount of weight, you must consume twice as many calories each day. You must reduce your daily calorie consumption by half to lose 10 pounds in two weeks.

Cutting your calories is the first step to losing 10 pounds in two weeks. Without calorie restriction, it's impossible to drop 10 pounds in two weeks. Furthermore, extra cardio might be beneficial. Increase your protein intake as well. Increase your calorie intake to burn fat in two weeks. Over 500 grams of protein per day is not recommended. If you're not receiving results within these parameters, you may want to explore adding another session.

Allow yourself some time to adjust if you are new to exercising out. Be consistent and rest between circuits. Make sure to do as many repetitions as you can, and limit yourself to 10 each exercise.

The secret to dropping 10 pounds in two weeks is to do it in this manner. You'll be well on your way to a healthier and fitter physique if you follow this advice. So don't sweat it; the exercise isn't the most essential thing. In only two weeks, you may drop up to ten pounds. Don't get carried away with the latest exercise or diet craze.

How to Lose 2 Weeks of Weight

Maintaining a healthy weight requires understanding how to lose weight in two weeks. A low-fat, low-carbohydrate diet is essential. Replace these items with more protein and veggies to reduce your consumption of these foods. This diet will assist you in losing weight and maintaining it. You may lose a few pounds every day if you follow a rigorous diet.

Consult a trained nutritionist or doctor if you haven't been able to shed any weight. A healthy food plan can assist you in losing weight swiftly. But first and foremost, you must understand your unique requirements and objectives. The pace at which you lose weight is determined by a variety of variables, including your overall health and daily exercise levels. It's advisable to think about your eating habits, since they might have an impact on how much weight you can lose.

Try one of the numerous fad diets available if you're wondering how to lose weight in 2 weeks. These diets claim rapid weight reduction, but reducing weight in this time frame necessitates a lifestyle change. Taking the time to prepare your meals and consuming nutritious foods can assist you in achieving your objectives. Remember that two weeks is a short period of time, and it's critical to make adjustments gradually. Finally, if you're serious about reducing weight, you must modify your lifestyle.

The most crucial aspect is to have faith in your ability to do the task. It's not impossible to lose weight, even if it's a challenging procedure. Maintaining a balanced diet and leading an active lifestyle might help you lose weight faster. Remember that if you want to lose a pound of fat, you'll need a 500-calorie deficit every day. And when you're attempting to reduce weight, that's precisely what you should concentrate on.

Without Exercise, How to Lose Weight in 2 Weeks

You've come to the correct site if you want to know how to lose weight in two weeks without exercising. It's simple to do, and the benefits will be seen in a week or two. But how can you extend the life of it? The finest ways for reducing weight rapidly will be discussed in this post. Calorie restriction is the key to reducing weight. Here are a few pointers to assist you in achieving your objective.

It's a terrific strategy to lose weight quickly if you change your diet once a week. However, you may find this time-consuming and annoying, and you may abandon your supper plans as a result. Without working out, you may drop a few pounds in two weeks by following to a few nutritious meals and a tight workout routine. It will also assist you in maintaining your weight loss. This will keep you from overindulging in bad meals, which may lead to future health issues.

You should increase the amount of healthy fats in your diet in addition to reducing calories. Working exercise is a fantastic method to reduce weight, but it is not the only option. Other techniques to enhance weight reduction in two weeks include drinking more water, cutting down on calories, and boosting your fat intake. If you're uncertain about a particular diet or activity regimen, you should seek medical guidance.

If you're serious about reducing weight, get advice from a doctor or nutritionist before beginning any activity or diet program. This is due to the fact that losing the required weight in two weeks will need a significant amount of work. Keep in mind that the aim is to lose at least 20 pounds, not just a couple!

To get the best results, make certain you have the right guidance and motivation. If you want a fast fix, the lifestyle described above may help you lose weight in a few of weeks.

Chapter Eight

Apple Cider Vinegar: Lose Weight in 2 Weeks

Drinking apple cider vinegar before a meal, according to one research, might help you lose weight in two weeks. Obese adults who used ACV on a regular basis dropped an average of 2.6 pounds, according to the study's findings. Although the effects of vinegar on the body are unknown, drinking it before meals may help to curb your hunger. This is an effective fat-burning supplement that you may take on a regular basis.

Improving satiety is critical for weight reduction success. You want to feel satisfied after you eat, therefore drinking apple cider vinegar can help you do that. It also prevents overeating by making you feel filled for longer. In a 2005 research, the amount of ACV that was beneficial when combined with carbohydrates was determined. It was shown that after eating a meal, people who drank the most ACV felt more content and carrier.

Another research found that giving rats apple cider vinegar before meals decreased their food intake, resulting in weight loss and decreased appetite. Despite the fact that this research was done on rats, it is vital to emphasize that no human studies have been done. The data were inconclusive, therefore the decision was made. The majority of the research included drinking apple cider vinegar as part of a healthy diet, with moderate outcomes. Check out my site for more information on how to lose weight using apple cider vinaigrette. It is low-cost and has been used in kitchens for thousands of years.

Apple cider vinegar may also help you eat less. Although it has been shown to reduce hunger and stomach upset, this natural weight loss aid does have some drawbacks. The drink's sole serious flaw is its awful flavor. This remedy's main drawback is that it may induce stomach pain. However, if you decide to give it a week, you will undoubtedly be pleased with the outcomes.

2 Week Diet Plan to Lose Weight

A weight-loss diet can be difficult but not impossible to follow. A two-week plan should aim for a one-to-two-pound weekly weight loss. You should eat 17,500 calories less than your maintenance calorie intake to lose five pounds in a week. If you make lifestyle changes to support your goal, a two-week diet is much more manageable. Learn how to get the best results from a two-week diet plan in this article.

This diet aims to help you lose two pounds in two weeks. The diet must be followed for at least six days, and three meals and two snacks must be consumed each day. It's not meant to be used for an extended period of time. Furthermore, the plan necessitates a lifestyle change if you want to lose even more weight. To put it another way, dieters who follow this plan can expect to lose up to 20 pounds in two weeks.

For various reasons, people seek to lose weight. Some people want to lose weight for the sake of being healthier, while others want to look good. While there are a variety of ways to lose weight, surgery and pills are not the most effective. Changing your lifestyle and eating habits are the best and healthiest ways to lose weight. You can lose 20 pounds in a month with a two-week diet plan. Before beginning a two-week diet plan, a number of factors should be considered.

Always seek advice from a qualified nutritionist or doctor before starting any diet plan. You could lose up to 20 pounds in two weeks depending on the weight loss program you choose. But keep in mind that losing weight quickly necessitates self-discipline and dedication. A diet that lasts longer than two weeks is not recommended. To keep your new figure, you must be willing to make lifestyle changes. This plan is a fantastic way to lose weight quickly if you're serious about losing weight.

Dietary discipline and a positive attitude are required for the two-week diet plan. While it is possible to lose up to 20 pounds in two weeks, a successful weight loss program will necessitate a change in lifestyle. This is not a long-term diet plan. It's best used for a short period of time when You must quickly lose a few pounds. Consume nutritious foods if you want to lose weight. A crash diet isn't the best choice if you're looking for a two-week diet plan that will help you lose weight quickly and safely. This is a diet plan that should only be followed for a few weeks. It is not advised to be followed for a long period of time, for example. If you want to lose 20 pounds, however, you should stick to a two-week plan.

The quickest way to lose weight is through a crash diet. In two weeks, you'll lose about half your body weight, but if you want more long-term results, a healthier diet is recommended. The majority of crash diets will result in you regaining the weight you lost, so choose your diet wisely. If you don't lose weight properly, your health isn't worth it. There are a few factors that make losing weight in two weeks difficult, but if you don't do it correctly, you won't achieve your goals.

If you want to lose weight in two weeks, you should speak with a nutritionist and a doctor. These programs are designed to help you lose a few pounds each week and can be extremely effective if followed properly. To keep the weight off for a long period of time, you'll need to be disciplined and self-disciplined.

Exercising to Lose Weight in Two Weeks

Cutting calories is one of the most effective ways to lose 20 pounds in two weeks. You lose weight by burning more calories than you consume. This entails consuming fewer calories. The easier it is to maintain your new weight, the more you cut back. But, if you don't exercise, how can you achieve this goal? Making lifestyle changes is the most efficient way to lose weight in two weeks.

By exercising every day, you can achieve your goal. However, if you want to lose 10 pounds in two weeks, you'll need to create a much larger deficit than you burn in a single week. Instead of 500 calories, you should aim for a deficit of 17,500 calories if you only want to lose five pounds per week. That's a significant amount of money to lose in a single week. Furthermore, to keep up with the daily calories you're consuming, you'll need to exercise more than you normally would. This will necessitate three daily workouts.

You should exercise at least three times per week to lose 10 pounds in two weeks, but never more. Workouts that demand your maximum energy should always be done. You can set your goals to lose 10 pounds in two weeks if you're serious about losing weight. Make sure you complete the exercises in three sets, with a minimum of ten to twelve reps per set.

Exercises that require you to expend a lot of energy while still working within your physical limitations are the best for losing weight. Performing these exercises can help you lose up to 10 pounds in two weeks. For each exercise, three sets of 10-12 reps are required, depending on the intensity. This is the most effective two-week weight-loss method. You should be able to lose up to 10 pounds in two weeks if you stick to these recommendations.

2 Week Meal Plan to Lose Weight

Simple, healthy foods should be included in the two-week menu plan. This diet is ideal for people who want to lose weight but don't know where to begin. Recipes, workouts, and challenges are all included in BetterMe's meal plan. You can relax and watch the magic happen once you've started the plan. The first step is to stock up on nutritious foods that can be stored in your refrigerator. Frozen vegetables, as well as protein and fiber-rich meals, can be found in the frozen section. Purchase root vegetables such as potatoes, carrots, apples, and other root vegetables.

Eating healthy meals will help you lose weight in two weeks. Protein and low-calorie carbohydrates should both be present in your meals. High-calorie foods and sugary drinks should be avoided because they will only cause you to gain weight. Fresh fruits and vegetables, rather than candy or snacks, should be part of your daily diet. If you're feeling peckish, you can even indulge in some treats like ice cream.

This simple plan will help you lose 5 pounds in two weeks.

The fact that your body adjusts quickly to a new routine is the main reason why losing weight in two weeks is difficult. This is why it's critical to lose weight gradually and make small daily adjustments. Smaller changes are easier to keep up with than larger ones, and you'll notice the difference sooner. Keep the new eating habits in mind and don't go overboard.

It's critical to remember to stock up on extra ingredients after you've started your two-week meal plan. This way, if you get unexpected company or your tastes change, you can quickly prepare a backup meal. To keep track of what you eat and where you need to buy it, use a calendar or spreadsheet. The planner will also keep track of the different ingredients you'll need for a variety of meals.

2 Week Meal Plans to Lose Weight

Making lifestyle changes is one method for losing weight in two weeks. Basic staples like fruits and vegetables are part of a proper two-week meal plan. Furthermore, a clean eating plan emphasizes minimally processed, fresh foods that are low in salt, saturated fat, and sugar. To add flavor and extend shelf life, avoid using artificial ingredients. Make sure you like the flavor of your food. You can lose as much weight as you want in a short period of time by sticking to a healthy eating plan.

Pumpkin flavoring is abundant during the fall season. For the winter, we eat more pumpkin-flavored foods and wear heavier sweaters. If you want to lose 10 pounds in two weeks, however, you'll need to burn more than five pounds per week. To achieve your goal, keep in mind that you must consume 17,500 calories less than your maintenance level. So aiming for a diet plan that allows you to cut your food intake in half would be beneficial.

A two-week meal plan emphasizes healthy eating in addition to promoting it. It motivates you to eat more vegetables and stay away from processed snacks. It's a quick and easy way to shed pounds in just two weeks. You will feel more energetic and energized as a result of the increased amount of energy and decreased cravings. You can easily lose four pounds in two weeks if you follow the directions carefully.

You must consult a qualified nutritionist or doctor before beginning your weight-loss program. You may be able to achieve your weight loss goals within two weeks, depending on your current health and underlying health conditions. How fast you lose weight is also determined by your body's needs and the amount of daily activity you engage in. Then, depending on your schedule, you should adjust the plan. If you stick to the plan for a minimum of three weeks, you can indulge in the occasional treat.

Weight Loss Pills for 2 Weeks

You should be wary of diet pills that claim to help you lose weight in two weeks. While some pills advertise themselves as the best, others may be a waste of time and money. Before buying a pill, it's critical to read the label and understand the ingredients. Inquire with the manufacturer if you have any questions about the item. Furthermore, read the instructions on the bottle if you want the best results.

You should be aware of a few key facts about diet pills. First and foremost, don't believe all of the hype surrounding them. Natural pills are not addictive, but they do have a few drawbacks. You may experience mild to moderate side effects depending on their functionality and formulation. Before you buy anything, double-check the ingredients. The ingredients should not harm your body and should not cause any negative reactions.

Next, look for stimulants in the diet pills. Caffeine or guarana are found in some pills, but they are ineffective. You should consult your doctor before taking a diet pill. Sugar or starch are present in some of them in high amounts. You should also look for artificial ingredients in the product. Even if you live a healthy lifestyle, you may struggle to lose weight in some cases.

Finally, check to see if the pill comes with a money-back guarantee. Most supplements come with money-back guarantees, allowing you to return the pills if you are unhappy with the results. To see if they're right for you, you should give them at least a month of testing. You will receive your money back due to the refund policy. You can always try them again for a full refund if you're still not losing weight after a month.

There are numerous options for losing weight in two weeks. For a few weeks or even a month, you can take a diet pill. Taking the pills for several weeks is the most common method. Then you must eat a nutritious diet rich in fruits and vegetables. You can lose weight in a week by eating a high-fiber diet. It will also keep you healthy and keep you from contracting diseases.

Chapter Nine

Weight Loss Plan in 2 Weeks

Cutting back on calories is the most effective way to lose weight in two weeks. You will gain weight if you consume more calories than you burn. Reduce your food intake and increase your daily physical activity to lose weight in two weeks. Making lifestyle changes is required to lose up to 20 pounds in two weeks. Furthermore, to keep your metabolism high, you should exercise on a regular basis.

It's difficult for most people to lose weight, which is why it's difficult. Hunger pangs are triggered by the stress hormone cortisol, which tells the body to store more fat. This is why it's so difficult to lose weight quickly. Fortunately, by eating well and staying active, you can make it easier on yourself. The key is to find a weight-loss plan that is healthy and effective for you. It works a lot better than a crash diet.

You must be disciplined when losing weight. This diet promises to help you lose 20 pounds in two weeks. While it isn't a long-term solution, it can assist you in losing a few pounds in preparation for special occasions. If you can't stick to your new eating habits, a diet plan that requires strict self-control can help you lose weight more quickly. This is a two-week weight-loss plan, not a long-term diet.

When it comes to losing weight, quick results are not the best option. It's neither secure nor long-term. While rapid weight loss is a great way to lose weight quickly, it is not a healthy way to lose body fat. Furthermore, it is neither sustainable nor conducive to a healthy lifestyle. You'll need to change your lifestyle because this diet isn't long-term sustainable.

If you want to lose weight quickly, you must first determine whether or not you can maintain a healthy lifestyle. If you're overweight, the best diet for you is one that allows you to indulge in your favorite foods. If you want to lose weight quickly, it's a good idea to live a healthy lifestyle, but it won't be healthy long term. It's also crucial to stick to the diet to avoid future health problems.

2 Week Workout at Home to Lose Weight

You must restrict your caloric intake to lose 20 pounds in two weeks. Cutting your food intake by 20% is a good starting point. It's also a good idea to limit your snacking. Your body will quickly adapt to the new routine, so take it slowly at first. The first few weeks will be much less difficult than you anticipate. Remember to exercise at least three times per week.

While exercising is an obvious way to lose weight, it's also important to limit your calorie intake and raise your heart rate. It's more difficult to burn over 2,000 calories per day, so start with a smaller calorie deficit and gradually increase your daily exercise. Incorporating healthy fats into your diet is also a good idea. You can lose 10 pounds in two weeks if you follow these guidelines.

Set a daily calorie deficit if you want to lose weight in 2 weeks. This is an excellent place to begin your quest for a slimmer, more toned body. Keep in mind, however, that losing a few pounds is easier than losing ten. The more calories you burn, the faster you will lose weight. Calculate your maintenance calorie intake to set a daily calorie budget. Then, to burn an additional 2,000 calories per day, incorporate some exercise into your daily routine.

Another important tip for slimming down: don't let stress stop you from losing weight. You are more likely to snack when you are stressed. Cortisol, a stress hormone, causes the body to store more fat, making it difficult to lose weight. To achieve your goal, it would be best if you could avoid stress. However, keep in mind that if you're stressed, you'll need to exercise more to stay on track with your fitness goals.

Tips Without Exercise, How to Lose Weight in 2 Weeks

Reduce your calorie intake if you want to lose weight in two weeks. Only by eating fewer calories than you burn will you be able to achieve this. If you're wondering how to do it, it's as simple as eating less. You might believe it's impossible, but it's true! Following are some suggestions:

To begin, you must restrict your liquid consumption. The only drinks that will not make you dizzy are water and unsweetened coffee, both of which contain more calories than water. However, alcohol is a widely consumed beverage. There are 125 calories in a 12-ounce latte with whole milk. Limiting alcohol consumption for two weeks is the best way to lose weight quickly. Make sure you account for your alcohol consumption when calculating your daily energy needs.

You should increase your protein intake in addition to calorie reduction. If you want to lose weight quickly, stick to a low-carb, high-protein, high-fat diet. This diet will only work if you consult a dietitian or a physician, as it may not be healthy for you. A balanced diet should include a wide variety of foods and provide all of the nutrients your body requires. Get plenty of sleep, drink plenty of water, and eat plenty of lean proteins and vegetables. You should eat healthy fats in addition to meeting your daily energy needs.

You'll lose between one and two pounds in two weeks if you stick to this plan. If you want to lose more weight in a short period of time, you should consider following a diet and exercise plan. While dieting alone can help you lose weight, it's not recommended unless you have a lot of it to lose. You should only try this strategy after that.

Tips 2 Week Workout to Lose Weight

Do you want to drop a few pounds in less than two weeks? Then you must understand that weight loss rates vary and are dependent on your individual body. Make sure you implement the necessary lifestyle changes to maximize your weight loss in two weeks. You can lose more weight in two weeks if you follow the advice above. To maximize weight loss, you can combine a healthy diet with an exercise plan. A few ideas will be provided in this article.

In order to lose weight, you must be willing to go on a calorie-restricted diet. In order to lose weight, you must be willing to give up some calories. Your diet should be well-balanced and tailored to your level of fitness. It would be ideal if you were adamant about sticking to your plan. Your health, level of daily activity, and dietary preferences will all play a role. Furthermore, your objectives must be attainable and realistic.

It's best if you kept a strict calorie deficit as well. You must create a calorie deficit greater than your current maintenance level to lose 10 pounds in two weeks. To put it another way, you should aim to burn over 2,000 calories per day. To accomplish this, you must plan your dietary intake as well as your workout routine in a balanced and systematic manner. You must be committed to your goal if you want to lose weight in two weeks. You'll have no trouble staying on track once you've committed to a healthier lifestyle.

Keep your focus on your goals. It is not easy to lose 10 pounds in two weeks. It necessitates a dedicated mindset as well as a high degree of discipline. Here are a few pointers to help you stay on track to meet your goal. So get started on a weight-loss workout routine right now. Remember to seek advice from a fitness professional and to stick to your goals. You'll be glad you took the time to do so. Just remember to have a good time and look after yourself.

CPSIA information can be obtained
at www.ICGtesting.com
Printed in the USA
LVHW061739090422
715792LV00009B/549